SMOOTHIES FOR WEIGHT GAIN

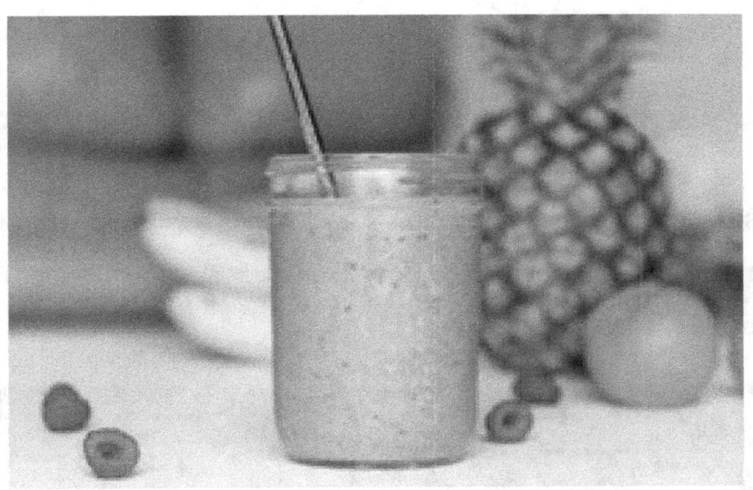

The ultimate guide to gaining weight the healthy way

Anna Moss

Copyright © 2023 by Anna Moss

All rights reserved

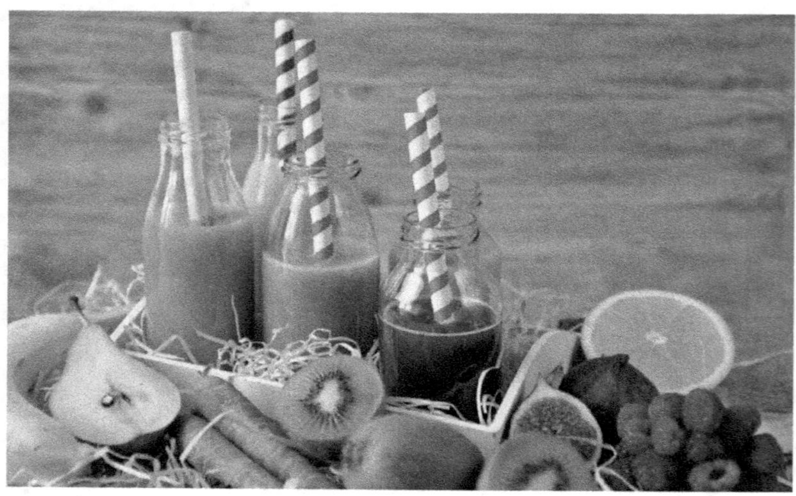

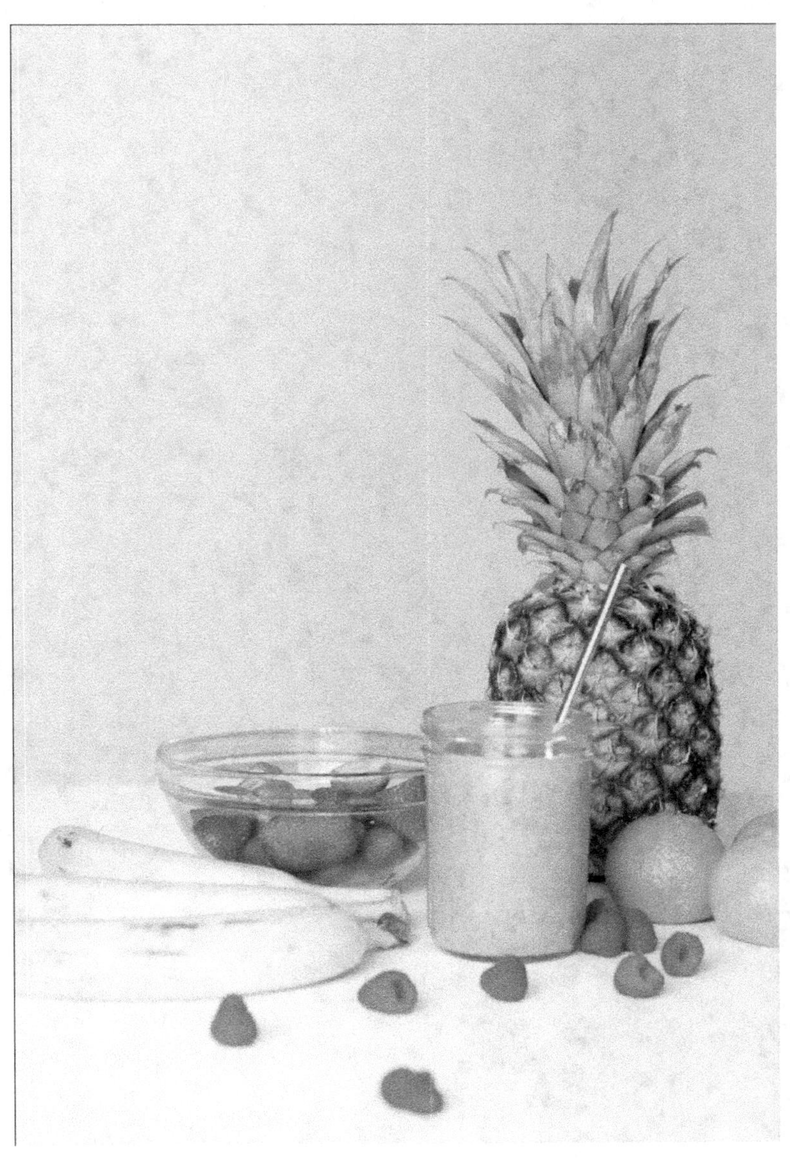

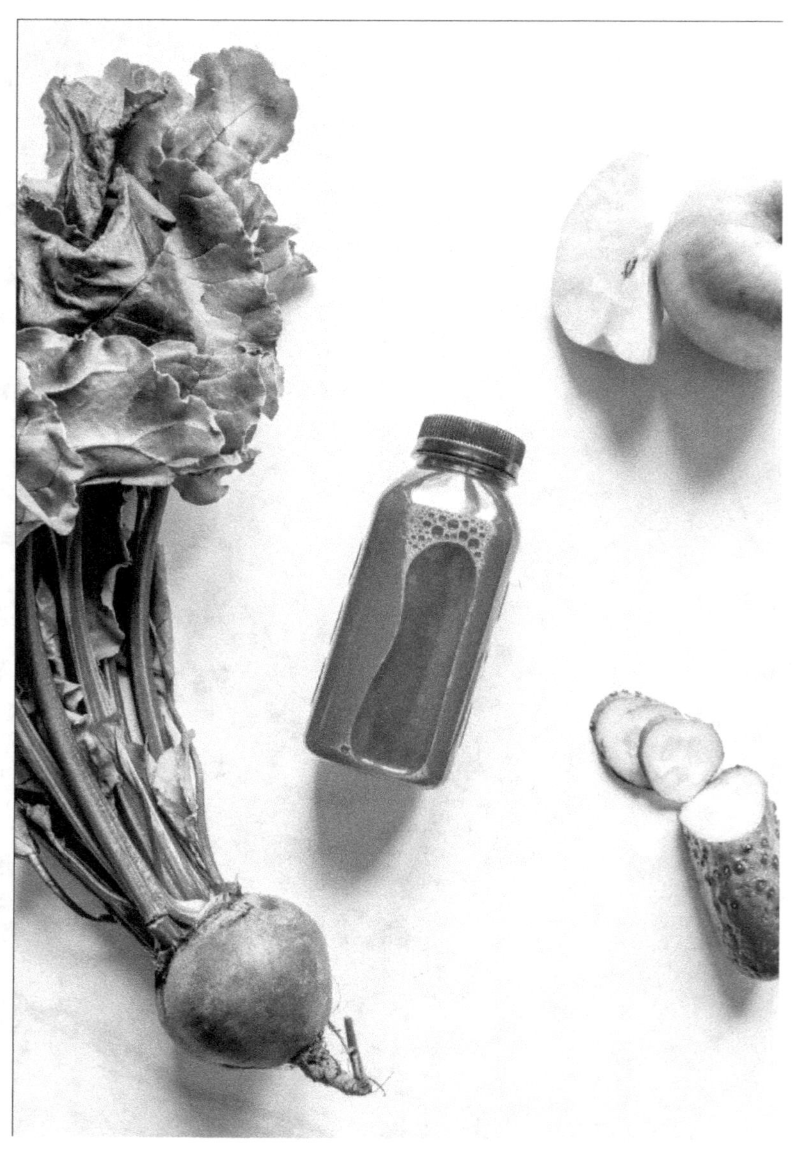

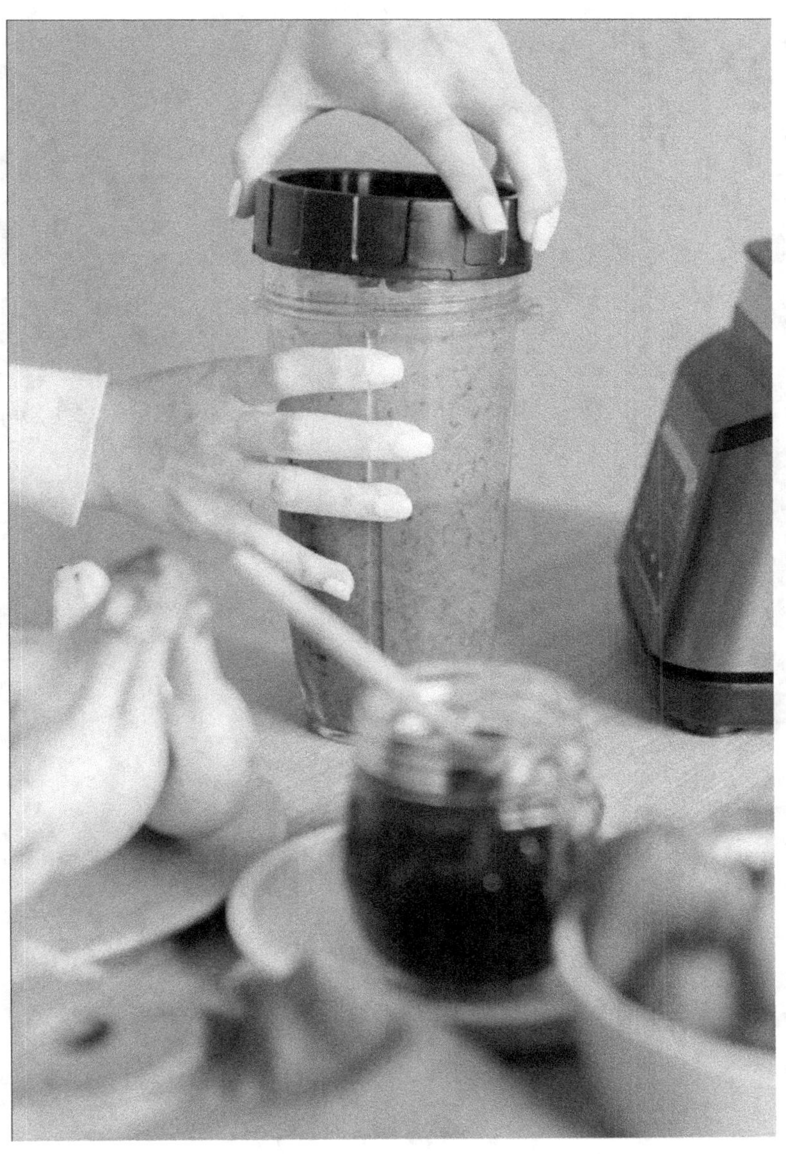

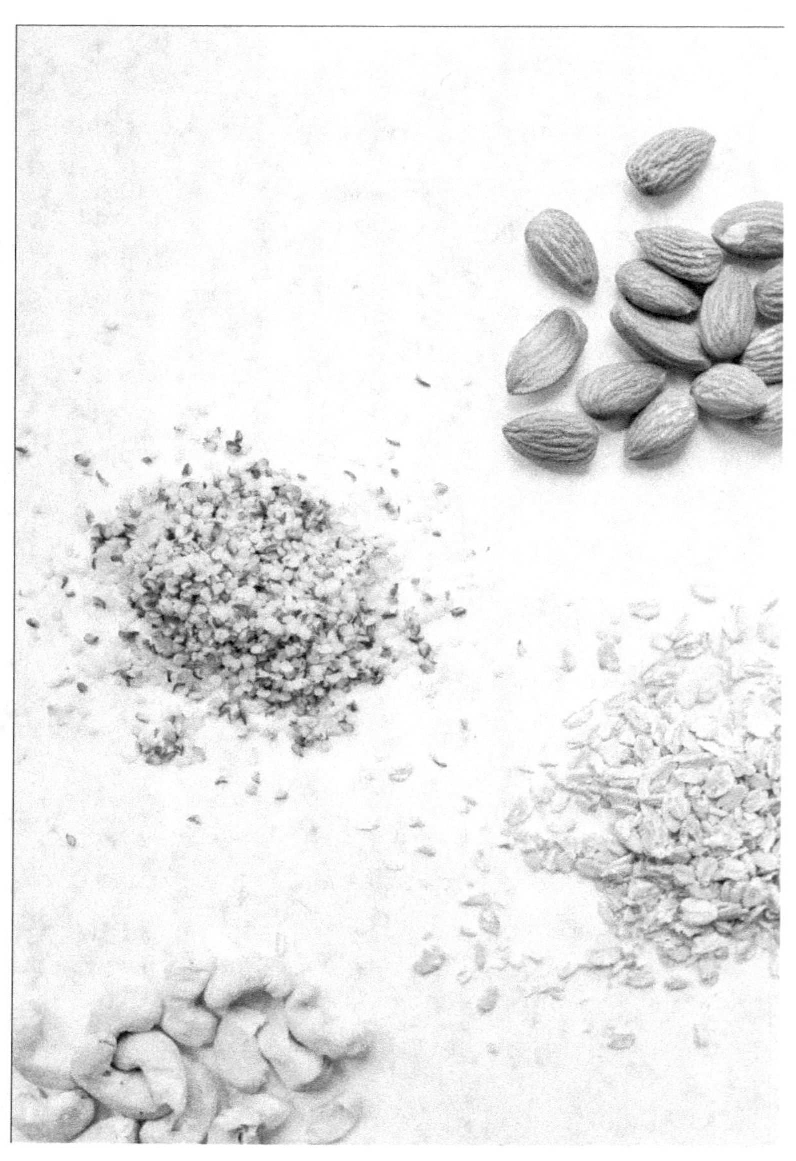

Table of Contents

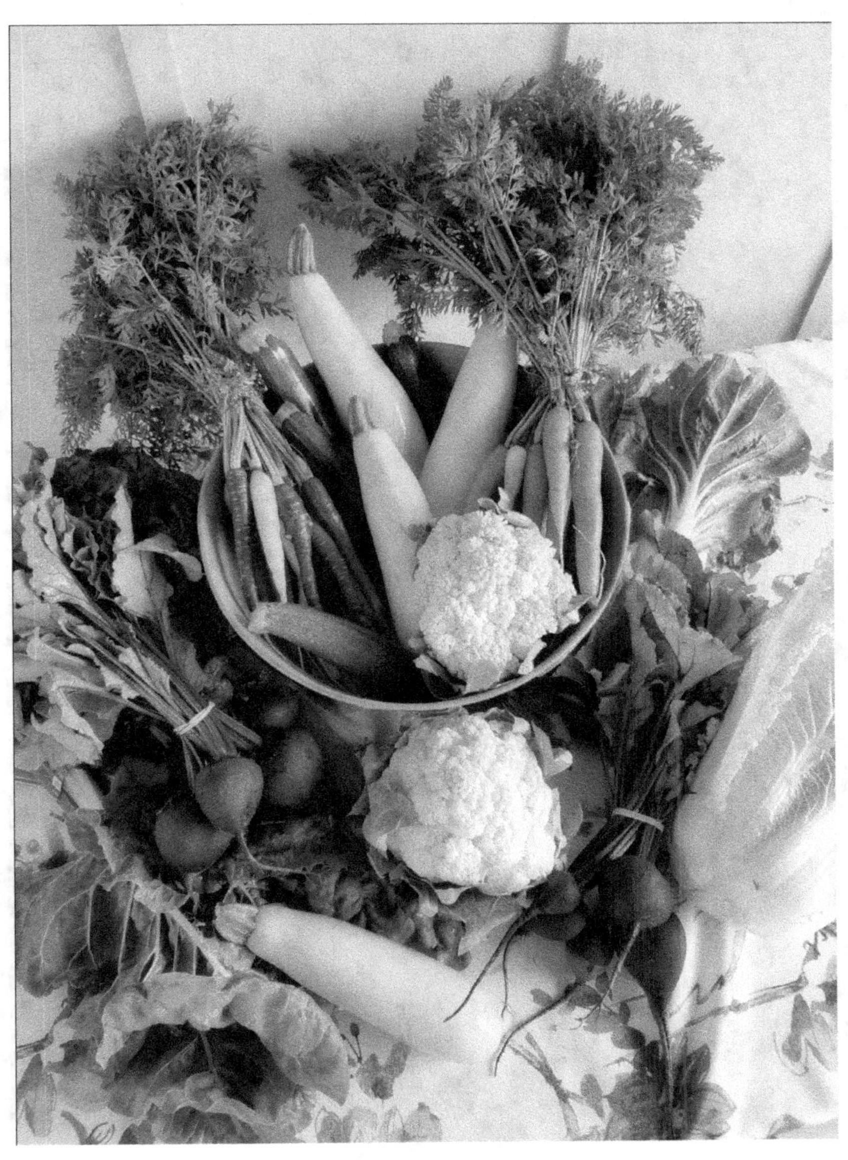

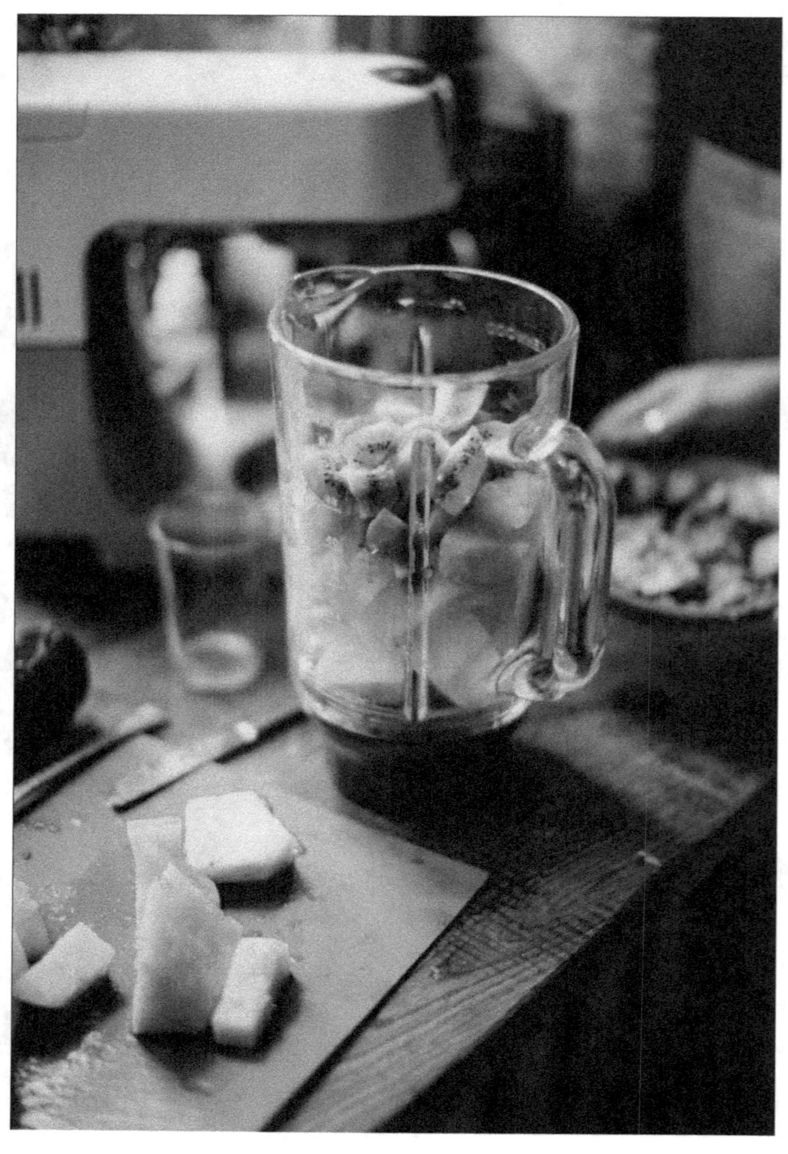

INTRODUCTION

Alex was a skinny guy who wanted to gain some weight, but was confused on how to do it. He asked his friends for advice and they all gave him the same advice - read smoothies for weight gain and follow the instructions.

Alex did, went to the store and bought himself some protein powder, blended fruits, and yogurt. He then started making smoothies every morning and drinking them for breakfast and lunch.

At first, he didn't see any results and felt discouraged. But then, after a few weeks, he started noticing a difference. He was feeling fuller after every meal and he noticed that his clothes were starting to fit a bit tighter.

Alex was ecstatic and kept drinking his smoothies every day. After a few months, he had gained 10 pounds and was feeling much better about himself.

He was amazed at how easy it was to gain weight with smoothies.

He was able to get the nutrients he needed without having to eat too much and without having to worry about gaining unhealthy fat.

Alex now drinks smoothies every day and loves the way he looks and feels. He's glad that he found such a simple and healthy way to gain weight.

It's no secret that gaining weight can be a struggle. Whether you're naturally thin, have a fast metabolism, or have lost weight due to an illness or lifestyle change, gaining weight can feel like an uphill battle.

Fortunately, there is a way to gain weight quickly and healthfully with smoothies. In this book, you'll learn how to make delicious and nutritious smoothies that will help you gain weight in a healthy, sustainable way. With an understanding of how each ingredient works together to increase your caloric intake, you'll be able to customize smoothies to meet your dietary needs and goals.

Get ready to take your weight gain journey to the next level with smoothies!

CHAPTER 1

Understanding smoothie weight gain

Smoothies for weight gain can be a great way to add extra calories to your diet, but it is important to understand what you're putting into your body.

Smoothies can help you gain weight, but you should also combine them with other healthy eating practices and regular exercise.

The key to gaining healthy weight with smoothies is to ensure that they include nutrient-rich ingredients. These should include fruits, nuts, and/or seeds, as well as sources of protein and healthy fats. For example, you might create a smoothie with a banana, some almond butter, and hemp seeds for a healthy, calorie-dense snack.

You may also consider adding protein powder to your smoothie for extra calories and protein. However, you should always check the ingredients list to ensure that the protein powder is made with a quality source of protein and doesn't contain a lot of added sugar or other unhealthy ingredients.

To ensure that you're getting the most out of your smoothie, make sure to drink it slowly and savor the flavors. This will help to keep you feeling full for longer and prevent you from overeating or snacking on unhealthy foods.

Finally, don't forget to stay hydrated. Drinking plenty of water throughout the day can help to keep your metabolism running smoothly and can also help to prevent overeating.

Benefits of smoothies for weight gain

Smoothies are a great way to gain weight in a healthy way. They are packed with healthy ingredients, such as fruits, vegetables, nuts, and seeds, which provide essential vitamins and minerals, as well as calories to help with weight gain.

Smoothies are convenient, easy to make, and can be customized to fit your individual nutritional needs. They also provide a great way to get extra protein, which is essential for building muscle.

Some of the benefits are:

1. Increased energy levels: Smoothies are a great source of energy and can help provide you with a burst of energy when you need it. This can help you to stay active and productive throughout the day, which can be beneficial for weight gain.

2. Improved digestion: Smoothies are easy to digest, which means that they can help to improve your digestive health and help you take in more nutrients from the ingredients in your smoothie. This can be beneficial for weight gain as you'll be able to get more of the essential nutrients that your body needs.

3. Variety of ingredients: Smoothies are a great way to get a variety of ingredients into your diet. You can add anything from fruits and vegetables to protein powders, nuts, seeds, and more to your smoothie, which can allow you to get a wider range of vitamins, minerals, and other essential nutrients into your diet, which can be beneficial for weight gain.

4. High in protein: Protein is essential for weight gain, and smoothies can be a great source of protein. You can add protein powders, nut butters, and other ingredients to your smoothie to ensure you're getting enough protein into your diet.

5. Balanced nutrition: Smoothies are a great way to get a balanced nutrition. You can add a variety of ingredients to your smoothie to ensure you're getting enough essential nutrients, vitamins, and minerals in your diet to fuel your body and help with weight gain.

6. Convenience: Smoothies are an incredibly convenient way to get the nutrition you need. You can make a smoothie in minutes, and you can take it with you on the go if you need to. This makes it easier to fit healthy eating into your busy lifestyle and ensure that you're getting the nutrition you need for weight gain.

7. Low in calories: Smoothies can be low in calories, which can be beneficial for those who are trying to gain weight. You can add healthy fats, such as avocado and nut butters, to your smoothie to increase the calorie content without compromising on the health benefits.

8. Healthy fats: Healthy fats are essential for weight gain, and smoothies are a great way to get them into your diet. You can add healthy fats, such as avocado, nut butters, and coconut oil, to your smoothie to increase the calorie content and get healthy fats into your diet.

9. High in fiber: Fiber is essential for weight gain, and smoothies can be a great way to get enough fiber into your diet. Adding ingredients such as chia seeds, flax seeds, and nuts to your smoothie can help to increase the fiber content, which can be beneficial for weight gain.

10. Easy to customize: Smoothies are incredibly easy to customize. You can add whatever ingredients you like to your smoothie to make it taste the way you like, and you can also adjust the calorie content to make it easier to gain weight.

Finally, smoothies are a great way to get in extra calories without feeling overly full or bloated. You can make a smoothie that is nutrient-dense and calorie-dense, but still easy to digest. This makes it easy to get in extra calories without feeling overly full or uncomfortable.

How to Manage Your Weight the Healthy Way

Maintaining a healthy lifestyle requires a healthy approach to weight management.

To get you started, think about the following ideas:

1. Eat a balanced diet that contains a variety of nutrient-dense foods to maintain a healthy weight. Get plenty of whole grains, lean proteins, fruits, veggies, and healthy fats in your diet.

2. Be active: Regular exercise is necessary to maintain a healthy weight. Exercise for at least 30 minutes.

3. Monitor your caloric intake: Monitoring your caloric intake may aid in weight management. Use a food-tracking software to help you stay on target.

4. Get adequate rest. Controlling appetite and energy levels requires sleep. If you can, aim for 7-8 hours of sleep each night.

5. Consume less added sugar: Added sugar is typically included in prepared foods and may contribute to weight gain. The amount of extra sugar you eat should be maintained to a minimum.

6. Hydrate: Drinking adequate water could make you feel full and reduce your craving for harmful foods. Make an effort to consume at least 8 glasses of water per day.

By following these recommendations, you can maintain a positive relationship with your weight. Remember to consult your doctor if you have any questions or concerns regarding your health or weight.

CHAPTER 2

Shopping for smoothie ingredients

Shopping for smoothie ingredients can be a fun and rewarding experience. Whether you are looking for something to make a quick breakfast or an afternoon snack, smoothies are a great option. With just a few ingredients, you can create a tasty and nutritious smoothie.

When shopping for smoothie ingredients, it is important to consider what type of smoothie you are making. Different ingredients are needed for different types of smoothies.

Here are some pointers to get you going:

1. Choose your base. The base for your smoothie will be your primary ingredient and will provide the majority of the flavor and texture. You can choose from a variety of different liquids such as water, milk, coconut water, and juices.

2. Select fruits and veggies. Fruits and vegetables are the heart of a smoothie and provide vitamins, minerals, and fiber. When choosing your ingredients, make sure to select a variety of colors to ensure that you are getting all of your daily nutrients.

3. Add healthy fats. Healthy fats such as nut butter, coconut oil, and avocado can add a creamy texture and provide essential fatty acids.

4. Choose your protein. Protein helps keep you full and can be added in the form of protein powder, Greek yogurt, or nuts and seeds.

5. Consider adding a superfood. Superfoods such as chia seeds, flaxseed, and acai are packed with antioxidants and can provide additional health benefits.

6. Choose a sweetener. If you want to add a little sweetness, you can choose from a variety of natural sweeteners such as honey, maple syrup, or dates.

By following these tips, you can easily shop for smoothie ingredients to make a delicious and nutritious smoothie. Enjoy!

CHAPTER 3

Basics of Smoothie Making

Smoothie making is a great way to get creative with your diet and a perfect way to pack a lot of nutrients into a single glass. If you're looking to learn the basics of smoothie making,

Here are the basics of smoothie making.

1. Choose your base. This is usually a liquid such as milk, yogurt, juice, or water. Depending on the type of smoothie you're making, you can choose dairy or non-dairy options.

2. Pick your fruit. Frozen or fresh fruit can be used, but frozen fruit will give your smoothie a thicker, creamier texture. Bananas are a great addition to most smoothies, as they help to add sweetness and creaminess.

3. Choose your add-ins. This could be anything from protein powder to nut butters, chia seeds, flax seeds, and more.

4. Add your flavourings. This can be anything from honey and maple syrup to cocoa powder and spices. 5. Blend it all together. Start by adding the liquid and then slowly add the other ingredients.

Blend until you reach your desired consistency. Once you have your smoothie made, you can enjoy it or take it on the go.

You can also add toppings such as nuts, granola, or fresh fruit for an extra special touch.

CHAPTER 4

Basic weight-gain smoothie recipes

A weight gain smoothie is an excellent way to get the extra calories needed to build muscle and gain weight. They are simple to make and can be varied to suit your taste and nutritional needs.

Here are a few basic weight-gain smoothie recipes to get you started.

1. Banana Coconut Smoothie: This smoothie is high in protein and healthy fats, making it ideal for weight gain. Combine 1 banana, 1 cup of coconut milk, 2 tablespoons of almond butter, and 1 tablespoon of honey in a blender. Blend until smooth and enjoy.

2. Peanut Butter and Jelly Smoothie: This smoothie is packed with protein, carbohydrates, and healthy fats. Combine 1 cup of almond milk, 2 tablespoons of peanut butter, 1 banana, 1 tablespoon of honey, and 1/4 cup of frozen berries in a blender. Blend until smooth and enjoy.

3. Chocolate & Oats Smoothie: This smoothie is high in protein and carbohydrates, making it great for gaining weight. Combine 1 cup of almond milk, 1 banana, 2 tablespoons of cocoa powder, 2 tablespoons of oats, and 1 tablespoon of honey in a blender. Blend until smooth and enjoy.

4. Blueberry & Avocado Smoothie: This smoothie is packed with healthy fats and protein, making it great for weight gain. Combine 1 cup of almond milk, 1/2 avocado, 1/2 cup of frozen blueberries, 2 tablespoons of almond butter, and 1 tablespoon of honey in a blender. Blend until smooth and enjoy.

These are just a few basic weight-gain smoothie recipes to get you started. You can get creative and use different fruits, nuts, seeds, and other healthy ingredients to make your own unique smoothie.

CHAPTER 5

Advanced weight-gain smoothie recipes

If you're looking to gain weight, you may find yourself searching for the best ways to do so. Eating healthy, nutrient-dense foods is important, and smoothies are a great way to get the nutrients you need in a convenient, delicious way.

Advanced weight-gain smoothie recipes can help you increase your calorie and nutrient intake, providing your body with the building blocks for healthy weight gain.

When it comes to making a weight-gain smoothie, there are a few key components to consider.

Start by choosing a base of either almond milk, coconut milk, cow's milk, or a plant-based milk alternative. Then, add a source of healthy fats such as peanut butter, avocado, or ground flaxseed.

These will help you increase your calorie intake while providing essential fatty acids that your body needs.

Next, add a complex carbohydrate such as oatmeal, oats, or quinoa. Complex carbohydrates are an important source of energy and provide essential vitamins and minerals.

You can also add a scoop of protein powder, such as whey or plant-based protein powder. Protein powder helps build and repair muscle and can also help you feel fuller for longer.

Finally, you can add some fruit or vegetables to your smoothie to provide essential vitamins, minerals, and antioxidants.

Bananas, mangoes, berries, and spinach are all great options. If you're looking for an even bigger calorie boost, you can add nuts, nut butters, or seeds for some extra healthy fats and protein.

Once you've chosen your ingredients, add them to your blender with some ice and blend until smooth. If your smoothie is too thick, add a bit of almond milk or water to thin it out.

Advanced weight-gain smoothie recipes can provide you with the calories and nutrients you need to gain weight in a healthy way.

Make sure to choose a variety of ingredients that provide healthy fats, complex carbohydrates, and protein to give your body the building blocks it needs to gain weight. With the right ingredients and a blender, you can make a delicious weight-gain smoothie in no time.

Weight gain smoothie recipes

1. Banana, Oats, and Almond Butter Smoothie

Ingredients:

- 1 banana

- 1/4 cup rolled oats

- 2 tablespoons almond butter

- 1 cup almond milk

- 1/2 teaspoon cinnamon

Instructions:

- Place all ingredients in a blender.

- Blend until smooth.

- Serve and enjoy!

2. Peanut Butter and Banana Smoothie

Ingredients:

- 1 banana

- 1 tablespoon peanut butter

- 1/2 cup plain Greek yogurt

- 1/4 cup milk

- 2 tablespoons honey

Instructions:

- Place all ingredients in a blender.

- Blend until smooth.

- Serve and enjoy!

3. Peanut Butter and Chocolate Protein Smoothie

Ingredients:

- 1 banana

- 1 tablespoon peanut butter

- 1 scoop chocolate protein powder

- 1 cup milk

- 2 tablespoons cocoa powder

Instructions:

- Place all ingredients in a blender.

- Blend until smooth.

- Serve and enjoy!

4. Oatmeal, Banana, and Almond Milk Smoothie

Ingredients:

- 1 banana

- 1/2 cup rolled oats

- 1 cup almond milk

- 1/2 teaspoon vanilla extract

- 2 tablespoons almond butter

Instructions:

- Place all ingredients in a blender.

- Blend until smooth.

- Serve and enjoy!

5. Strawberry, Banana, and Chia Seeds Smoothie

Ingredients:

- 1 banana

- 1/2 cup frozen strawberries

- 1 cup almond milk

- 2 tablespoons chia seeds

- 1/2 teaspoon vanilla extract

Instructions:

- Place all ingredients in a blender.

- Blend until smooth.

- Serve and enjoy!

6. Coconut, Banana, and Greek Yogurt Smoothie

Ingredients:

- 1 banana

- 1/4 cup coconut milk

- 1/2 cup Greek yogurt

- 2 tablespoons honey

- 1 teaspoon coconut flakes

Instructions:

- Place all ingredients in a blender.

- Blend until smooth.

- Serve and enjoy!

7. Peanut Butter and Jelly Smoothie

Ingredients:

- 1 banana

- 1 tablespoon peanut butter

- 1/4 cup jelly

- 1 cup milk

- 2 tablespoons honey

Instructions:

- Place all ingredients in a blender.

- Blend until smooth.

- Serve and enjoy!

8. Chocolate, Banana, and Coconut Smoothie

Ingredients:

- 1 banana

- 2 tablespoons cocoa powder

- 1/4 cup coconut milk

- 1 cup almond milk

- 2 tablespoons honey

Instructions:

- Place all ingredients in a blender.

- Blend until smooth.

- Serve and enjoy!

9. Avocado, Banana, and Almond Milk Smoothie

Ingredients:

- 1 banana

- 1/2 avocado

- 1 cup almond milk

- 2 tablespoons honey

- 1/2 teaspoon vanilla extract

Instructions:

- Place all ingredients in a blender.

- Blend until smooth.

- Serve and enjoy!

10. Peanut Butter, Banana, and Oats Smoothie

Ingredients:

- 1 banana

- 1 tablespoon peanut butter

- 1/4 cup rolled oats

- 1 cup almond milk

- 2 tablespoons honey

Instructions:

- Place all ingredients in a blender.

- Blend until smooth.

- Serve and enjoy!

11. Banana and Almond Butter Smoothie

Ingredients:

- 1 banana

- 2 tablespoons almond butter

- 1/2 cup almond milk

- 1/2 teaspoon cinnamon

- 2 tablespoons honey

Instructions:

- Place all ingredients in a blender.

- Blend until smooth.

- Serve and enjoy!

12. Apple, Banana, and Oats Smoothie

Ingredients:

- 1 banana

- 1/2 apple, peeled and cored

- 1/4 cup rolled oats

- 1 cup almond milk

- 2 tablespoons honey

Instructions:

- Place all ingredients in a blender.

- Blend until smooth.

- Serve and enjoy!

13. Peanut Butter, Banana, and Honey Smoothie

Ingredients:

- 1 banana

- 1 tablespoon peanut butter

- 1/2 cup almond milk

- 2 tablespoons honey

- 1/2 teaspoon vanilla extract

Instructions:

- Place all ingredients in a blender.

- Blend until smooth.

- Serve and enjoy!

14. Peanut Butter and Banana Smoothie Bowl

Ingredients:

- 1 banana

- 1 tablespoon peanut butter

- 1/2 cup almond milk

- 1/4 cup Greek yogurt

- 1/4 cup granola

Instructions:

- Place all ingredients except granola in a blender.

- Blend until smooth.

- Pour into a bowl and top with granola.

- Serve and enjoy!

15. Chocolate, Banana, and Almond Milk Smoothie

Ingredients:

- 1 banana

- 1 tablespoon cocoa powder

- 1/2 cup almond milk

- 2 tablespoons honey

- 1/2 teaspoon vanilla extract

Instructions:

- Place all ingredients in a blender.

- Blend until smooth.

- Serve and enjoy!

16. Banana, Oats, and Coconut Milk Smoothie

Ingredients:

- 1 banana

- 1/4 cup rolled oats

- 1/2 cup coconut milk

- 2 tablespoons honey

- 1/2 teaspoon coconut flakes

Instructions:

- Place all ingredients in a blender.

- Blend until smooth.

- Serve and enjoy!

17. Blueberry, Banana, and Almond Milk Smoothie

Ingredients:

- 1 banana

- 1/2 cup frozen blueberries

- 1 cup almond milk

- 2 tablespoons honey

- 1/2 teaspoon vanilla extract

Instructions:

- Place all ingredients in a blender.

- Blend until smooth.

- Serve and enjoy!

18. Peanut Butter, Banana, and Greek Yogurt Smoothie

Ingredients:

- 1 banana

- 1 tablespoon peanut butter

- 1/2 cup Greek yogurt

- 1/2 cup almond milk

- 2 tablespoons honey

Instructions:

- Place all ingredients in a blender.

- Blend until smooth.

- Serve and enjoy!

19. Peanut Butter, Banana, and Coconut Smoothie

Ingredients:

- 1 banana

- 1 tablespoon peanut butter

- 1/4 cup coconut milk

- 1 cup almond milk

- 2 tablespoons honey

Instructions:

- Place all ingredients in a blender.

- Blend until smooth.

- Serve and enjoy!

20. Strawberry, Banana, and Coconut Milk Smoothie

Ingredients:

- 1 banana

- 1/2 cup frozen strawberries

- 1/4 cup coconut milk

- 1/2 cup almond milk

- 2 tablespoons honey

Instructions:

- Place all ingredients in a blender.

- Blend until smooth.

- Serve and enjoy!

21. Chocolate, Peanut Butter, and Banana Smoothie

Ingredients:

- 1 banana

- 1 tablespoon cocoa powder

- 1 tablespoon peanut butter

- 1 cup almond milk

- 2 tablespoons honey

Instructions:

- Place all ingredients in a blender.

- Blend until smooth.

- Serve and enjoy!

22. Peanut Butter, Banana, and Oats Smoothie Bowl

Ingredients:

- 1 banana

- 1 tablespoon peanut butter

- 1/4 cup rolled oats

- 1 cup almond milk

- 2 tablespoons honey

- 1/4 cup granola

Instructions:

- Place all ingredients except granola in a blender.

- Blend until smooth.

- Pour into a bowl and top with granola.

- Serve and enjoy!

23. Apple, Banana, and Almond Milk Smoothie

Ingredients:

- 1 banana

- 1/2 apple, peeled and cored

- 1/2 cup almond milk

- 2 tablespoons honey

- 1/2 teaspoon cinnamon

Instructions:

- Place all ingredients in a blender.

- Blend until smooth.

- Serve and enjoy!

24. Peanut Butter and Banana Smoothie Bowl

Ingredients:

- 1 banana

- 1 tablespoon peanut butter

- 1/2 cup almond milk

- 1/4 cup Greek yogurt

- 1/4 cup granola

Instructions:

- Place all ingredients except granola in a blender.

- Blend until smooth.

- Pour into a bowl and top with granola.

- Serve and enjoy!

25. Chocolate, Peanut Butter, and Banana Smoothie Bowl

Ingredients:

- 1 banana

- 1 tablespoon cocoa powder

- 1 tablespoon peanut butter

- 1/2 cup almond milk

- 2 tablespoons honey

- 1/4 cup granola

Instructions:

- Place all ingredients except granola in a blender.

- Blend until smooth.

- Pour into a bowl and top with granola.

- Serve and enjoy!

26. Almond Butter, Banana, and Coconut Milk Smoothie

Ingredients:

- 1 banana

- 2 tablespoons almond butter

- 1/4 cup coconut milk

- 1 cup almond milk

- 2 tablespoons honey

Instructions:

- Place all ingredients in a blender.

- Blend until smooth.

- Serve and enjoy!

27. Peanut Butter, Banana, and Oats Smoothie

Ingredients:

- 1 banana

- 1 tablespoon peanut butter

- 1/4 cup rolled oats

- 1 cup almond milk

- 2 tablespoons honey

Instructions:

- Place all ingredients in a blender.

- Blend until smooth.

- Serve and enjoy!

28. Banana, Oats, and Coconut Milk Smoothie

Ingredients:

- 1 banana

- 1/4 cup rolled oats

- 1/2 cup coconut milk

- 2 tablespoons honey

- 1/2 teaspoon cinnamon

Instructions:

- Place all ingredients in a blender.

- Blend until smooth.

- Serve and enjoy!

29. Strawberry, Banana, and Greek Yogurt Smoothie

Ingredients:

- 1 banana

- 1/2 cup frozen strawberries

- 1/2 cup Greek yogurt

- 1/2 cup almond milk

- 2 tablespoons honey

Instructions:

- Place all ingredients in a blender.

- Blend until smooth.

- Serve and enjoy!

30. Banana, Oats, and Almond Milk Smoothie Bowl

Ingredients:

- 1 banana

- 1/4 cup rolled oats

- 2 tablespoons almond butter

- 1 cup almond milk

- 2 tablespoons honey

- 1/4 cup granola

Instructions:

- Place all ingredients except granola in a blender.

- Blend until smooth.

- Pour into a bowl and top with granola.

- Serve and enjoy!

31. Banana and Peanut Butter Smoothie

Ingredients:

- 1 banana

- 1 tablespoon peanut butter

- 1/2 cup almond milk

- 2 tablespoons honey

- 1/2 teaspoon vanilla extract

Instructions:

- Place all ingredients in a blender.

- Blend until smooth.

- Serve and enjoy!

32. Avocado, Banana, and Greek Yogurt Smoothie

Ingredients:

- 1 banana

- 1/2 avocado

- 1/2 cup Greek yogurt

- 1/2 cup almond milk

- 2 tablespoons honey

Instructions:

- Place all ingredients in a blender.

- Blend until smooth.

- Serve and enjoy!

33. Peanut Butter and Banana Smoothie Bowl

Ingredients:

- 1 banana

- 1 tablespoon peanut butter

- 1/2 cup almond milk

- 1/4 cup Greek yogurt

- 1/4 cup granola

Instructions:

- Place all ingredients except granola in a blender.

- Blend until smooth.

- Pour into a bowl and top with granola.

- Serve and enjoy!

34. Peanut Butter, Banana, and Almond Milk Smoothie

Ingredients:

- 1 banana

- 1 tablespoon peanut butter

- 1/2 cup almond milk

- 2 tablespoons honey

- 1/2 teaspoon cinnamon

Instructions:

- Place all ingredients in a blender.

- Blend until smooth.

- Serve and enjoy!

35. Chocolate, Peanut Butter, and Banana Smoothie

Ingredients:

- 1 banana

- 1 tablespoon cocoa powder

- 1 tablespoon peanut butter

- 1 cup almond milk

- 2 tablespoons honey

Instructions:

- Place all ingredients in a blender.

- Blend until smooth.

- Serve and enjoy!

36. Apple, Banana, and Greek Yogurt Smoothie

Ingredients:

- 1 banana

- 1/2 apple, peeled and cored

- 1/2 cup Greek yogurt

- 1/2 cup almond milk

- 2 tablespoons honey

Instructions:

- Place all ingredients in a blender.

- Blend until smooth.

- Serve and enjoy!

37. Peanut Butter, Banana, and Coconut Milk Smoothie

Ingredients:

- 1 banana

- 1 tablespoon peanut butter

- 1/4 cup coconut milk

- 1 cup almond milk

- 2 tablespoons honey

Instructions:

- Place all ingredients in a blender.

- Blend until smooth.

- Serve and enjoy!

38. Banana, Oats, and Almond Milk Smoothie Bowl

Ingredients:

- 1 banana

- 1/4 cup rolled oats

- 2 tablespoons almond butter

- 1 cup almond milk

- 2 tablespoons honey

- 1/4 cup granola

Instructions:

- Place all ingredients except granola in a blender.

- Blend until smooth.

- Pour into a bowl and top with granola.

- Serve and enjoy!

39. Chocolate, Banana, and Coconut Milk Smoothie

Ingredients:

- 1 banana

- 2 tablespoons cocoa powder

- 1/4 cup coconut milk

- 1 cup almond milk

- 2 tablespoons honey

Instructions:

- Place all ingredients in a blender.

- Blend until smooth.

- Serve and enjoy!

40. Peanut Butter, Banana, and Oats Smoothie Bowl

Ingredients:

- 1 banana

- 1 tablespoon peanut butter

- 1/4 cup rolled oats

- 1 cup almond milk

- 2 tablespoons honey

- 1/4 cup granola

Instructions:

- Place all ingredients except granola in a blender.

- Blend until smooth.

- Pour into a bowl and top with granola.

- Serve and enjoy!

41. Strawberry and Banana Smoothie

Ingredients:

- 1 banana

- 1/2 cup frozen strawberries

- 1 cup almond milk

- 2 tablespoons honey

- 1/2 teaspoon vanilla extract

Instructions:

- Place all ingredients in a blender.

- Blend until smooth.

- Serve and enjoy!

42. Peanut Butter, Banana, and Almond Milk Smoothie

Ingredients:

- 1 banana

- 1 tablespoon peanut butter

- 1/2 cup almond milk

- 2 tablespoons honey

- 1/2 teaspoon cinnamon

Instructions:

- Place all ingredients in a blender.

- Blend until smooth.

- Serve and enjoy!

43. Apple, Banana, and Coconut Milk Smoothie

Ingredients:

- 1 banana

- 1/2 apple, peeled and cored

- 1/4 cup coconut milk

- 1 cup almond milk

- 2 tablespoons honey

Instructions:

- Place all ingredients in a blender.

- Blend until smooth.

- Serve and enjoy!

44. Banana, Oats, and Almond Butter Smoothie Bowl

Ingredients:

- 1 banana

- 1/4 cup rolled oats

- 2 tablespoons almond butter

- 1 cup almond milk

- 2 tablespoons honey

- 1/4 cup granola

Instructions:

- Place all ingredients except granola in a blender.

- Blend until smooth.

- Pour into a bowl and top with granola.

- Serve and enjoy!

45. Chocolate, Peanut Butter, and Banana Smoothie Bowl

Ingredients:

- 1 banana

- 1 tablespoon cocoa powder

- 1 tablespoon peanut butter

- 1/2 cup almond milk

- 2 tablespoons honey

- 1/4 cup granola

Instructions:

- Place all ingredients except granola in a blender.

- Blend until smooth.

- Pour into a bowl and top with granola.

- Serve and enjoy!

46. Blueberry, Banana, and Greek Yogurt Smoothie

Ingredients:

- 1 banana

- 1/2 cup frozen blueberries

- 1/2 cup Greek yogurt

- 1/2 cup almond milk

- 2 tablespoons honey

Instructions:

- Place all ingredients in a blender.

- Blend until smooth.

- Serve and enjoy!

47. Banana, Oats, and Coconut Milk Smoothie Bowl

Ingredients:

- 1 banana

- 1/4 cup rolled oats

- 1/2 cup coconut milk

- 2 tablespoons honey

- 1/4 cup granola

Instructions:

- Place all ingredients except granola in a blender.

- Blend until smooth.

- Pour into a bowl and top with granola.

- Serve and enjoy!

48. Avocado, Banana, and Almond Milk Smoothie

Ingredients:

- 1 banana

- 1/2 avocado

- 1 cup almond milk

- 2 tablespoons honey

- 1/2 teaspoon vanilla extract

Instructions:

- Place all ingredients in a blender.

- Blend until smooth.

- Serve and enjoy!

49. Coconut, Banana, and Greek Yogurt Smoothie

Ingredients:

- 1 banana

- 1/4 cup coconut milk

- 1/2 cup Greek yogurt

- 2 tablespoons honey

- 1 teaspoon coconut flakes

Instructions:

- Place all ingredients in a blender.

- Blend until smooth.

- Serve and enjoy!

50. Carrot Cake Smoothie:

Ingredients:

- 1 banana

- 2 tablespoons of peanut butter

- 1/2 cup almond milk

- 2 tablespoons of cocoa powder

- 1 tablespoons honey

Instructions:

- Place all ingredients in a blender.

- Blend until smooth.

- Serve and enjoy!

CHAPTER 6

Smoothie preparation tips

Smoothies are a great way to get your daily dose of fruits and vegetables, as well as a tasty treat. Making a smoothie can be easy and fun, but there are a few things to keep in mind to make sure your smoothie comes out delicious every time.

To make the ideal smoothie, follow these suggestions.

1. Choose your ingredients wisely. Start with a base like milk, yogurt, or almond milk. Then, add a combination of fruits and vegetables. Berries are a great choice since they are full of antioxidants and add sweetness to the smoothie. Also, don't forget to add some healthy fats like nut butter or avocado for added creaminess.

2. Add some liquid. This will help make the smoothie easier to blend and will also add some extra flavor. You can use water, juice, or even coconut water.

3. Add protein. Protein helps to make the smoothie more filling and can also help to keep your blood sugar levels stable. You can add some protein powder or nut butter to your smoothie.

4. Use frozen ingredients. Frozen fruits and veggies will help make your smoothie thick and creamy. Plus, it will also help keep your smoothie cold for a longer period of time.

5. Don't overfill your blender. The more ingredients you add, the more difficult it can be to blend everything together. Try to fill your blender no more than two-thirds full.

6. Start blending on a lower speed and then increase it. This will help to prevent splashing and will also make sure everything is properly blended together.

7. Add some sweetness. If your smoothie needs a little bit of sweetness, try adding a natural sweetener like honey, maple syrup, or dates.

8. Drink it right away. Smoothies are best when they're freshly made, so make sure to drink it as soon as possible.

Making a smoothie can be a great way to get your daily dose of fruits and vegetables, as well as a tasty treat. Following these tips will help ensure that your smoothie comes out delicious every time. Enjoy!

CHAPTER 7

Common Smoothie Ingredients

Smoothies are a delicious and nutritious way to get a boost any time of day. Whether you're trying to eat healthier or just want to make a tasty treat, smoothies are a great choice. The best part is that you can customize them to your taste and dietary needs. To make a good smoothie, you need to start with the right ingredients. Here's a look at some of the most common smoothie ingredients and why they make a great addition to your smoothie.

Fruits: Fresh or frozen fruit is an essential part of any smoothie. Fruits are a great source of natural sweetness, vitamins, and minerals. Plus, they make your smoothie look and taste great. Popular fruits for smoothies include bananas, strawberries, blueberries, mangoes, and pineapples.

Vegetables: Vegetables are often overlooked in smoothies, but they add a lot of nutrition and flavor.

Try adding green leafy vegetables like spinach and kale, as well as carrots, beets, and sweet potato.

Yogurt: Yogurt is a great source of protein and can help make your smoothie creamy and thick. Greek yogurt is a great choice for adding protein, but any yogurt will do.

Milk: Milk is another great way to make your smoothie creamy and thick. You can use any type of milk, from cow's milk to plant-based milks like almond, coconut, or oat.

Nut Butter: Nut butter is a great source of healthy fats and can make your smoothie even creamier. Popular choices include almond butter, peanut butter, and cashew butter.

Honey: Honey is a great natural sweetener and can help balance out the flavour of your smoothie. Moreover, it is a fantastic antioxidant source.

Seeds: Seeds like chia, flax, and hemp are a great way to add healthy fats, fiber, and protein to your smoothie. They're also a great source of omega-3 fatty acids.

These are just a few of the most common smoothie ingredients. You can also add things like protein powder, fresh herbs, and spices to your smoothie to make it even more nutritious and flavourful.

Try out various combinations to see which one works best for you.. With the right ingredients, you can enjoy a delicious and nutritious smoothie any time of day.

CONCLUSION

The reader has been given a thorough review of the numerous ways that smoothies can be utilized to gain weight in a healthy and sustainable way in The Smoothie for Weight Gain Book.

The emphasis on the numerous nutritional advantages of preparing smoothies has equipped readers with the information and resources necessary to make wise choices regarding their weight-gain endeavors.

With this information, readers can progress in a safe, wholesome, and pleasurable manner toward their targeted weight goal. As with any weight-gain regimen, it's crucial to pay attention to your body's signals and modify your smoothie recipes as necessary.

Readers may rest easy knowing they are on the right path to achieving their desired weight gain objectives by creating a balanced and healthy food plan and utilizing the various advantages that smoothies offer.

Overall, those trying to gain weight in a healthy and sustainable way have found the Smoothie for Weight Growth Book to be an important resource.

By equipping readers with the essential information and resources, readers may now get the most out of their smoothie-making experience and take advantage of all its advantages.

With this, we hope that the material in this book has been helpful to readers and that they have been able to effectively achieve their intended weight gain objectives.